Mediterranean [Recipes for E

Super-Easy and Tasty Meat anc ⌐ Recipes to Improve Your Skills and Boost Your Taste

Fern Bullock

Table of Contents

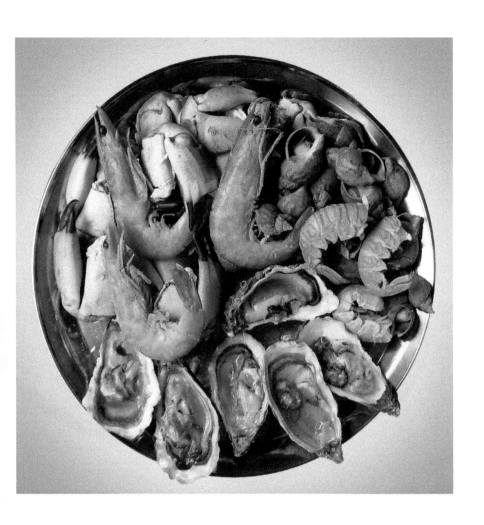

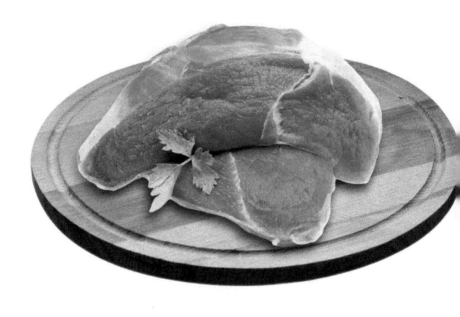

Salsa Bowls

Prep time: 10 minutes I **Cooking time:** 10 minutes I

Servings: 4

Ingredients:

- 1 tablespoon avocado oil
- 1 cup red bell peppers, cubed
- 1 pound cauliflower florets
- 1 red onion, chopped
- 3 tablespoons salsa
- 2 tablespoons cheddar, shredded
- 2 tablespoons coconut cream

Directions:

1. Heat up a pan with the oil over medium-high heat, add the onion and peppers, and sauté for 2 minutes.
2. Add the cauliflower and the other ingredients, toss, cook for 8 minutes more, divide into bowls and serve.

Nutrition facts per serving: calories 114, fat 5.5, fiber 4.3, carbs 12.7, protein 6.7

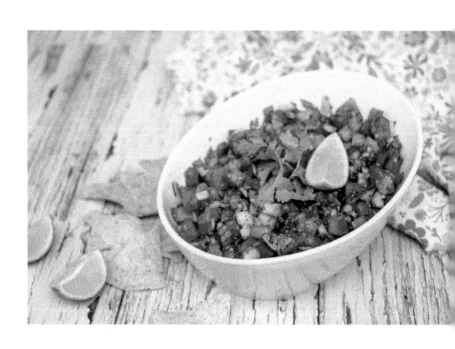

Yogurt Salmon Salad

Prep time: 5 minutes I **Cooking time:** 0 minutes I

Servings: 4

Ingredients:

- 1 cup smoked salmon, flaked
- 1 tablespoon lime zest, grated
- 1 tablespoon lime juice
- 3 tablespoons Greek yogurt
- 1 cup baby spinach
- 1 teaspoon capers, drained and chopped
- 1 red onion, chopped
- A pinch of black pepper
- 1 tablespoon chives, chopped

Directions:

1. In a bowl, combine the salmon with lime zest, lime juice and the other ingredients, toss and serve cold for lunch.

Nutrition facts per serving: calories 61, fat 1.9, fiber 1, carbs 5, protein 6.8

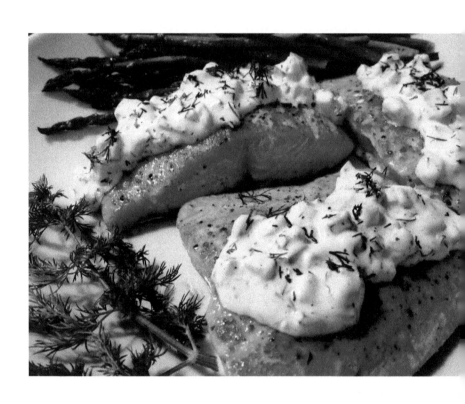

Mozzarella Chicken Mix

Prep time: 10 minutes I **Cooking time:** 20 minutes I
Servings: 4

Ingredients:

- 1 tablespoon olive oil
- 1 pound chicken breast, skinless, boneless and cubed
- ½ pound kale, torn
- 2 cherry tomatoes, halved
- 1 yellow onion, chopped
- ½ cup chicken stock
- ¼ cup mozzarella, shredded

Directions:

1. Heat up a pan with the oil over medium heat, add the chicken and the onion and brown for 5 minutes.
2. Add the kale and the other ingredients except the mozzarella, toss, and cook for 12 minutes more.
3. Sprinkle the cheese on top, cook the mix for 2-3 minutes, divide between plates and serve for lunch.

Nutrition facts per serving: calories 231, fat 6.5, fiber 2.7, carbs 11.4, protein 30.9

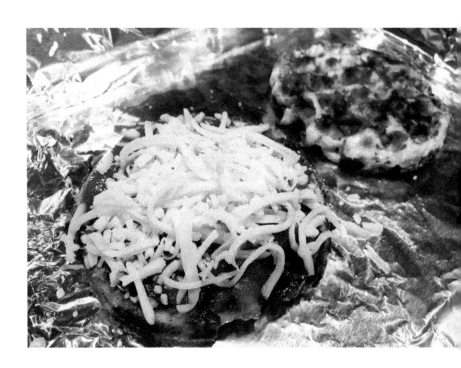

Salmon with Olives and Arugula Salad

Prep time: 10 minutes I **Cooking time:** 0 minutes I

Servings: 4

Ingredients:

- 6 ounces smoked salmon, cubed
- 1 tablespoon balsamic vinegar
- 1 tablespoon olive oil
- 2 shallots, chopped
- ½ cup black olives, pitted and halved
- 2 cups baby arugula
- A pinch of black pepper

Directions:

1. In a bowl, combine the salmon with the shallots and the other ingredients, toss and keep in the fridge for 10 minutes before serving for lunch.

Nutrition facts per serving: calories 113, fat 8, fiber 0.7, carbs 2.3, protein 8.8

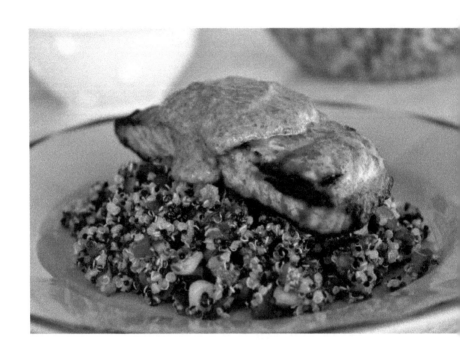

Shrimp and Carrots Salad

Prep time: 5 minutes I **Cooking time:** 10 minutes I

Servings: 4

Ingredients:

- 1 tablespoon olive oil
- 1 pound shrimp, peeled and deveined
- 1 tablespoon basil pesto
- 1 cup baby arugula
- 1 yellow onion, chopped
- 1 cucumber, sliced
- 1 cup carrots, shredded
- 1 tablespoon cilantro, chopped

Directions:

1. Heat up a pan with the oil over medium heat, add the onion and carrots, stir and cook for 3 minutes.
2. Add the shrimp and the other ingredients, toss, cook for 7 minutes more, divide into bowls and serve.

Nutrition facts per serving: calories 200, fat 5.6, fiber 1.8, carbs 9.9, protein 27

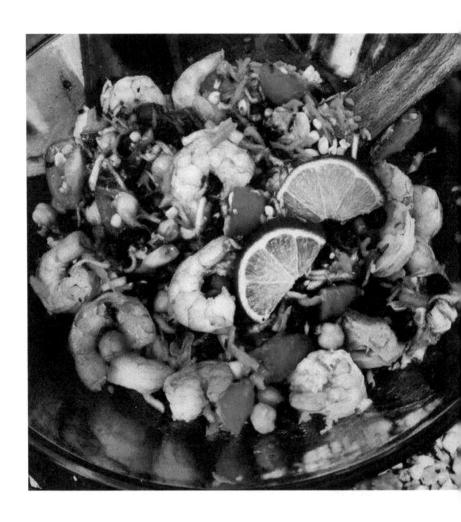

Turkey Tortillas

Prep time: 10 minutes I **Cooking time:** 3 minutes I
Servings: 2

Ingredients:

- 2 whole wheat tortillas
- 2 teaspoons mustard
- 2 teaspoons mayonnaise (hand-made)
- 1 turkey breast, skinless, boneless and cut into strips
- 1 tablespoons olive oil
- 1 red onion, chopped
- 1 red bell peppers, cut into strips
- 1 green bell pepper, cut into strips
- ¼ cup mozzarella, shredded

Directions:

1. Heat up a pan with the oil over medium heat, add the meat and the onion and brown for 5 minutes
2. Add the peppers, toss and cook for 10 minutes more.
3. Arrange the tortillas on a working surface, divide the turkey mix on each, also divide the mayo, mustard and the cheese, wrap and serve for lunch.

Nutrition facts per serving: calories 342, fat 11.6 fiber 7.7, carbs 39.5, protein 21.9

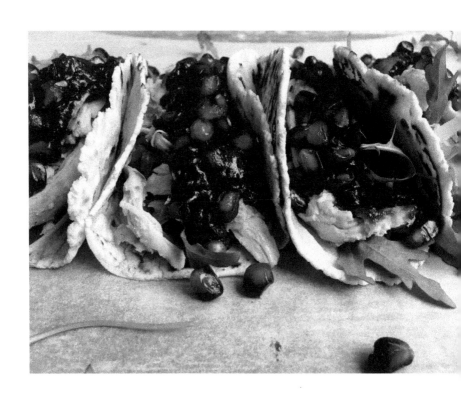

Black Beans Soup

Prep time: 5 minutes I **Cooking time:** 35 minutes I
Servings: 4

Ingredients:

- 2 teaspoons olive oil
- 2 garlic cloves, minced
- 1 pound black beans, soaked overnight and drained
- 1 yellow onion, chopped
- 2 tomatoes, cubed
- 1 teaspoon sweet paprika
- 1 quart chicken stock
- 2 tablespoons parsley, chopped

Directions:

1. Heat up a pot with the oil over medium-high heat, add the garlic and the onion, stir and sauté for 5 minutes.
2. Add the beans and the other ingredients except the parsley, stir, bring to a simmer and cook for 30 minutes.
3. Add the parsley, stir, divide the soup into bowls and serve.

Nutrition facts per serving: calories 87, fat 2.7, fibe 5.5, carbs 14, protein 4.1

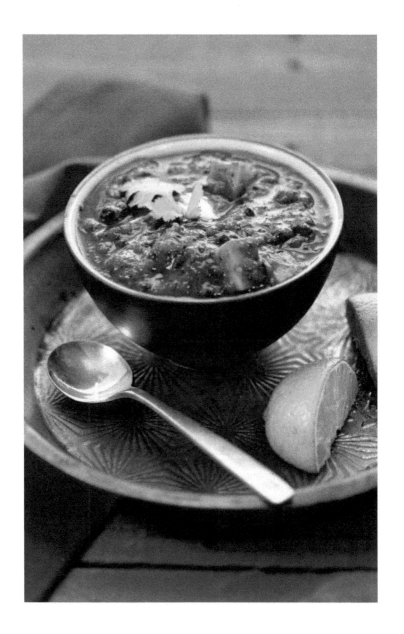

Mint Spinach Salad

Prep time: 5 minutes I **Cooking time:** 0 minutes I

Servings: 4

Ingredients:

- 2 tablespoon balsamic vinegar
- 2 tablespoons mint, chopped
- A pinch of black pepper
- 1 avocado, peeled, pitted and sliced
- 4 cups baby spinach
- 1 cup black olives, pitted and halved
- 1 cucumber, sliced
- 1 tablespoon olive oil

Directions:

1. In a salad bowl, combine the avocado with the spinach and the other ingredients, toss and serve for lunch.

Nutrition facts per serving: calories 192, fat 17.1, fiber 5.7, carbs 10.6, protein 2.7

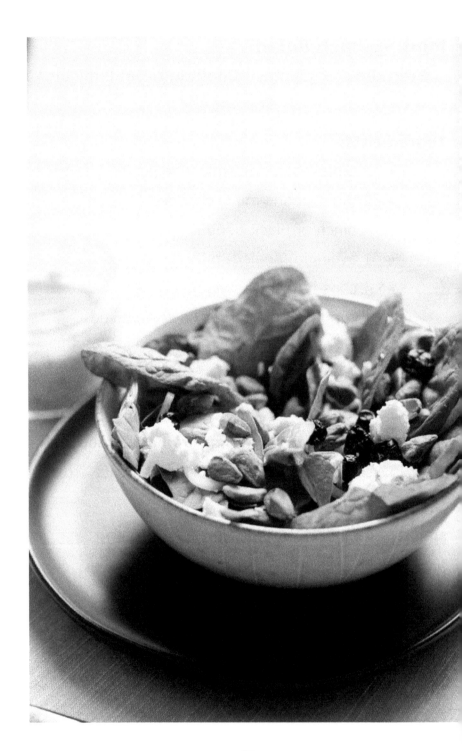

Beef Pan

Prep time: 5 minutes I **Cooking time:** 20 minutes I **Servings:** 4

Ingredients:

- 1 pound beef, ground
- ½ cup yellow onion, chopped
- 1 tablespoon olive oil
- 1 cup zucchini, cubed
- 2 garlic cloves, minced
- 14 ounces tomatoes, chopped
- 1 teaspoon Italian seasoning
- ¼ cup parmesan, shredded
- 1 tablespoon chives, chopped
- 1 tablespoon cilantro, chopped

Directions:

1. Heat up a pan with the oil over medium heat, add the garlic, onion and the beef and brown for 5 minutes.
2. Add the rest of the ingredients, toss, cook for 15 minutes more, divide into bowls and serve for lunch.

Nutrition facts per serving: calories 276, fat 11.3, fiber 1.9, carbs 6.8, protein 36

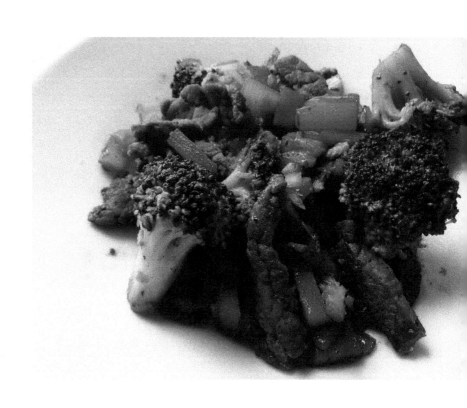

Thyme Beef

Prep time: 10 minutes I **Cooking time:** 25 minutes I

Servings: 4

Ingredients:

- ½ pound beef, ground
- 3 tablespoons olive oil
- 1 and ¾ pounds red potatoes, peeled and roughly cubed
- 1 yellow onion, chopped
- 2 teaspoons thyme, dried
- 1 cup tomatoes, chopped
- A pinch of black pepper

Directions:

1. Heat up a pan with the oil over medium-high heat, add the onion and the beef, stir and brown for 5 minutes.
2. Add the potatoes and the rest of the ingredients, toss, bring to a simmer, cook for 20 minutes more, divide into bowls and serve for lunch.

Nutrition facts per serving: calories 216, fat 14.5, fiber 5.2, carbs 40.7, protein 22.2

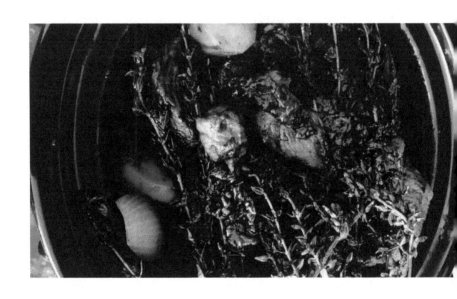

Pork Soup

Prep time: 10 minutes I **Cooking time:** 25 minutes I **Servings:** 4

Ingredients:

- 1 tablespoon olive oil
- 1 red onion, chopped
- 1 pound pork stew meat, cubed
- 1 quart beef stock
- 1 pound carrots, sliced
- 1 cup tomato puree
- 1 tablespoon cilantro, chopped

Directions:

1. Heat up a pot with the oil over medium-high heat, add the onion and the meat and brown for 5 minutes.
2. Add the rest of the ingredients except the cilantro, bring to a simmer, reduce heat to medium, and boil the soup for 20 minutes.
3. Ladle into bowls and serve for lunch with the cilantro sprinkled on top.

Nutrition facts per serving: calories 354, fat 14.6, fiber 4.6, carbs 19.3, protein 36

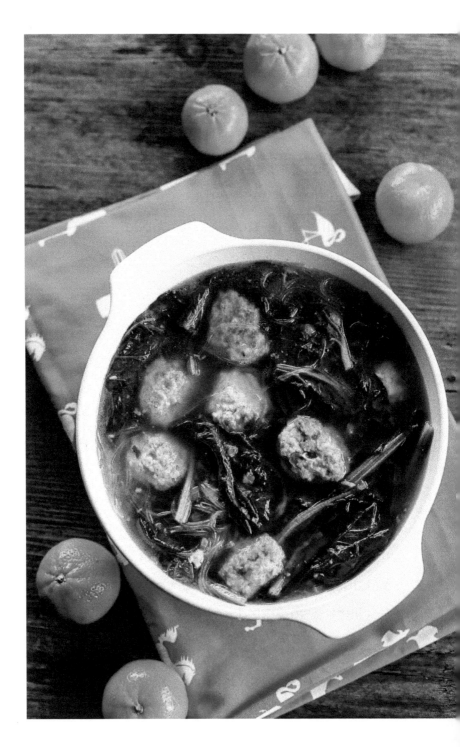

Shrimp and Corn Salad

Prep time: 5 minutes I **Cooking time:** 7 minutes I

Servings: 4

Ingredients:

- 1 cup corn
- 1 endive, shredded
- 1 cup baby spinach
- 1 pound shrimp, peeled and deveined
- 2 garlic cloves, minced
- 1 tablespoon lime juice
- 2 cups strawberries, halved
- 2 tablespoons olive oil
- 2 tablespoons balsamic vinegar
- 1 tablespoon cilantro, chopped

Directions:

1. Heat up a pan with the oil over medium-high heat, add the garlic and brown for 1 minute. Add the shrimp and lime juice, toss and cook for 3 minutes on each side.
2. In a salad bowl, combine the shrimp with the corn, endive and the other ingredients, toss and serve for lunch.

Nutrition facts per serving: calories 260, fat 9.7, fiber 2.9, carbs 16.5, protein 28

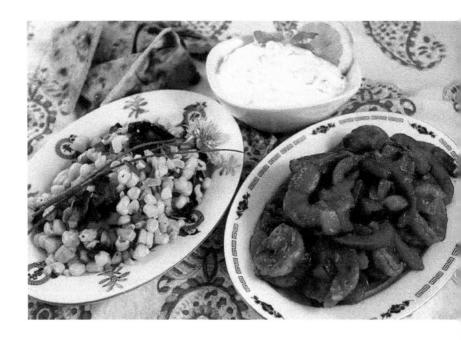

Raspberry Shrimp Salad

Prep time: 5 minutes I **Cooking time:** 10 minutes I

Servings: 4

Ingredients:

- 1 pound green beans, trimmed and halved
- 2 tablespoons olive oil
- 2 pounds shrimp, peeled and deveined
- 1 tablespoon lemon juice
- 2 cups cherry tomatoes, halved
- ¼ cup raspberry vinegar
- A pinch of black pepper

Directions:

1. Heat up a pan with the oil over medium-high heat, add the shrimp, toss and cook for 2 minutes.
2. Add the green beans and the other ingredients, toss, cook for 8 minutes more, divide into bowls and serve for lunch.

Nutrition facts per serving: calories 385, fat 11.2, fiber 5, carbs 15.3, protein 54.5

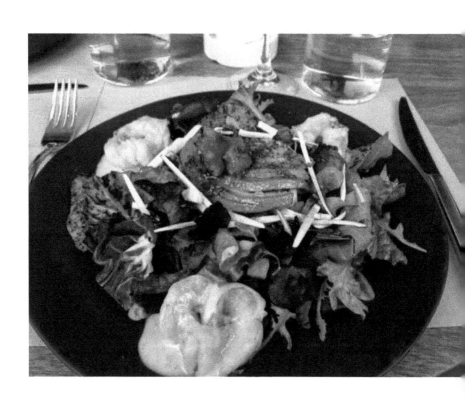

Tacos

Prep time: 10 minutes I **Cooking time:** 10 minutes I

Servings: 2

Ingredients:

- 4 whole wheat taco shells
- 1 tablespoon light mayonnaise
- 1 tablespoon salsa
- 1 tablespoon mozzarella, shredded
- 1 tablespoon olive oil
- 1 red onion, chopped
- 1 tablespoon cilantro, chopped
- 2 cod fillets, boneless, skinless and cubed
- 1 tablespoon tomato puree

Directions:

1. Heat up a pan with the oil over medium heat, add the onion, stir and cook for 2 minutes.
2. Add the fish and tomato puree, toss gently and cook for 5 minutes more.
3. Spoon this into the taco shells, also divide the mayo, salsa and the cheese and serve for lunch.

Nutrition facts per serving: calories 466, fat 14.5, fiber 8, carbs 56.6, protein 32.9

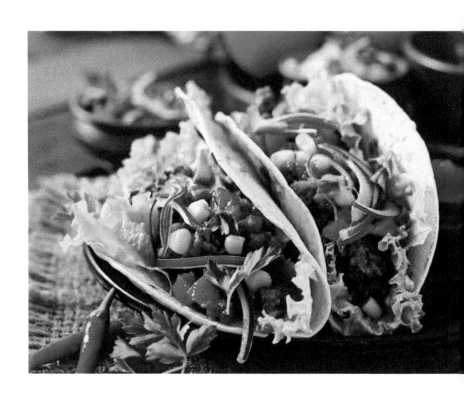

Zucchini and Carrot Cakes

Prep time: 10 minutes I **Cooking time:** 10 minutes I

Servings: 4

Ingredients:

- 1 yellow onion, chopped
- 2 zucchinis, grated
- 2 tablespoons almond flour
- 1 egg, whisked
- 1 garlic clove, minced
- A pinch of black pepper
- 1/3 cup carrot, shredded
- 1/3 cup cheddar, grated
- 1 tablespoon cilantro, chopped
- 1 teaspoon lemon zest, grated
- 2 tablespoons olive oil

Directions:

1. In a bowl, combine the zucchinis with the garlic, onion and the other ingredients except the oil, stir well and shape medium cakes out of this mix.
2. Heat up a pan with the oil over medium-high heat, add the zucchini cakes, cook for 5 minutes on each side, divide between plates and serve with a side salad.

Nutrition facts per serving: calories 271, fat 8.7, fiber 4, carbs 14.3, protein 4.6

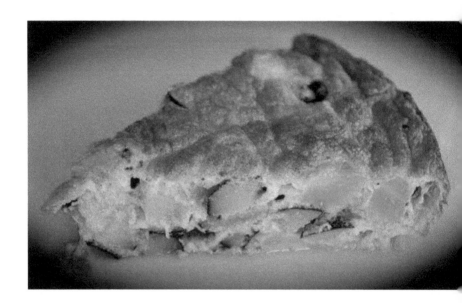

Chickpeas Stew

Prep time: 10 minutes I **Cooking time:** 20 minutes I
Servings: 4

Ingredients:

- 1 tablespoon olive oil
- 1 yellow onion, chopped
- 2 teaspoons chili powder
- 14 ounces chickpeas, cooked
- 14 ounces tomatoes, cubed
- 1 cup chicken stock
- 1 tablespoon cilantro, chopped
- A pinch of black pepper

Directions:

1. Heat up a pot with the oil over medium-high heat, add the onion and chili powder, stir and cook for 5 minutes.
2. Add the chickpeas and the other ingredients, toss, cook for 15 minutes over medium heat, divide into bowls and serve for lunch.

Nutrition facts per serving: calories 299, fat 13.2, fiber 4.7, carbs 17.2, protein 8.1

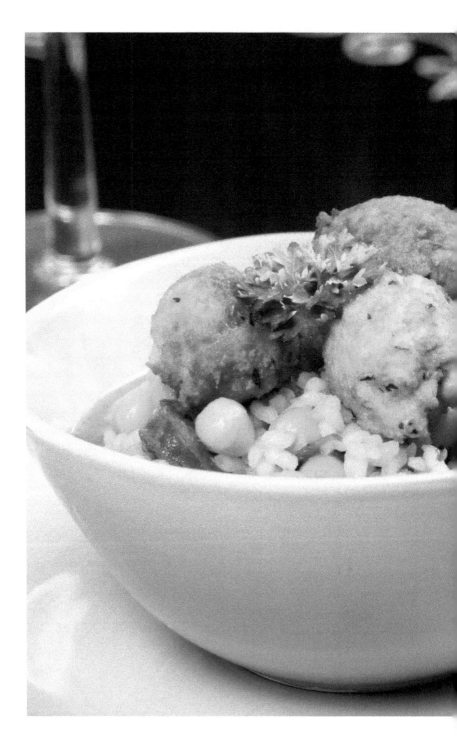

Chicken Salad

Prep time: 10 minutes I **Cooking time:** 0 minutes I
Servings: 4

Ingredients:

- 1 tablespoon olive oil
- A pinch of black pepper
- 2 rotisserie chicken, skinless, boneless, shredded
- 1 pound cherry tomatoes, halved
- 1 red onion, chopped
- 4 cups baby spinach
- ¼ cup walnuts, chopped
- ½ teaspoon lemon zest, grated
- 2 tablespoons lemon juice

Directions:

1. In a salad bowl, combine the chicken with the tomato and the other ingredients, toss and serve for lunch.

Nutrition facts per serving: calories 349, fat 8.3, fiber 5.6, carbs 16.9, protein 22.8

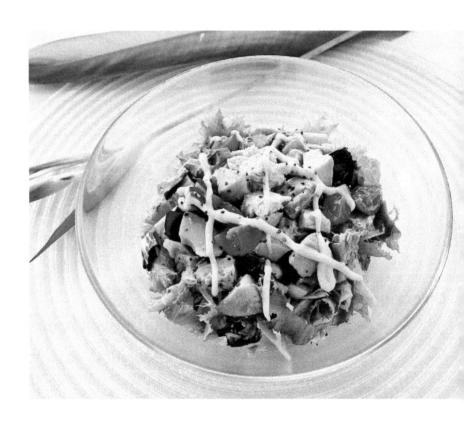

Warm Asparagus Salad

Prep time: 10 minutes I **Cooking time:** 20 minutes I
Servings: 4

Ingredients:

- 3 garlic cloves, minced
- 2 tablespoons olive oil
- 1 red onion, chopped
- 3 carrots, sliced
- ½ cup chicken stock
- 2 cups baby spinach
- 1 pound asparagus, trimmed and halved
- 1 red bell pepper, cut into strips
- 1 yellow bell pepper, cut into strips
- 1 green bell pepper, cut into strips
- A pinch of black pepper

Directions:

1. Heat up a pan with the oil over medium-high heat, add the onion and the garlic, stir and sauté for 2 minutes.
2. Add the asparagus and the other ingredients except the spinach, toss, and cook for 15 minutes.
3. Add the spinach, cook everything for 3 minutes more, divide into bowls and serve for lunch.

Nutrition facts per serving: calories 221, fat 11.2 fiber 3.4, carbs 14.3, protein 5.9

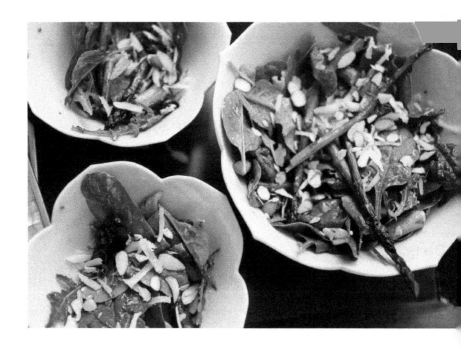

Beef Stew

Prep time: 10 minutes I **Cooking time:** 1 hour and 20 minutes I **Servings:** 4

Ingredients:

- 1 pound beef stew meat, cubed
- 1 cup tomato sauce
- 1 cup beef stock
- 1 tablespoon olive oil
- 1 yellow onion, chopped
- ¼ teaspoon hot sauce
- 1 teaspoon onion powder
- 1 teaspoon garlic powder
- 1 tablespoon cilantro, chopped

Directions:

1. Heat up a pot with the oil over medium-high heat, add the meat and the onion, stir and brown for 5 minutes.
2. Add the tomato sauce and the rest of the ingredients, bring to a simmer and cook over medium heat for 1 hour and 15 minutes.
3. Divide into bowls and serve for lunch.

Nutrition facts per serving: calories 487, fat 15.3, fiber 5.8, carbs 56.3, protein 15

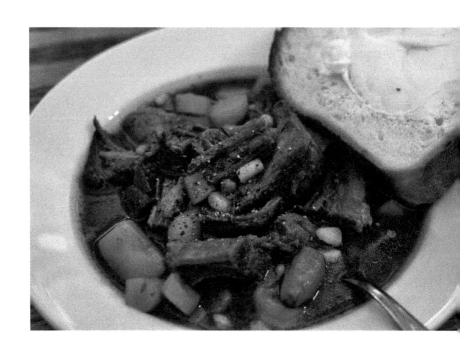

Rosemary Pork Chops

Prep time: 5 minutes I **Cooking time:** 8 hours and 10 minutes I **Servings:** 4

Ingredients:

- 4 pork chops
- 1 tablespoon olive oil
- 2 shallots, chopped
- 1 pound white mushrooms, sliced
- ½ cup beef stock
- 1 tablespoon rosemary, chopped
- ¼ teaspoon garlic powder
- 1 teaspoon sweet paprika

Directions:

1. Heat up a pan with the oil over medium-high heat, add the pork chops and the shallots, toss, brown for 10 minutes and transfer to a slow cooker.
2. Add the rest of the ingredients, put the lid on and cook on Low for 8 hours.
3. Divide the pork chops and mushrooms between plates and serve for lunch.

Nutrition facts per serving: calories 349, fat 24, fiber 5.6, carbs 46.3, protein 17.5

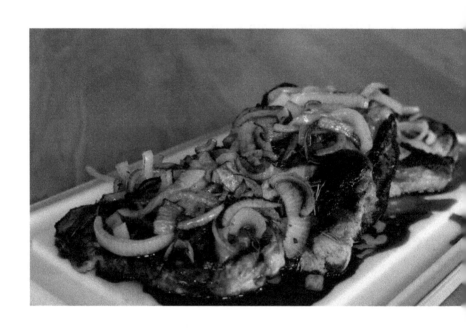

Shrimp, Arugula and Coriander Salad

Prep time: 10 minutes I **Cooking time:** 8 minutes I

Servings: 4

Ingredients:

- 1 tablespoon olive oil
- 1 red onion, sliced
- 1 pound shrimp, peeled and deveined
- 2 cups baby arugula
- 1 tablespoon balsamic vinegar
- 1 tablespoon lemon juice
- 1 tablespoon coriander, chopped
- A pinch of black pepper

Directions:

1. Heat up a pan with the oil over medium heat, add the onion, stir and sauté for 2 minutes.
2. Add the shrimp and the other ingredients, toss, cook for 6 minutes, divide into bowls and serve for lunch.

Nutrition facts per serving: calories 341, fat 11.5, fiber 3.8, carbs 17.3, protein 14.3

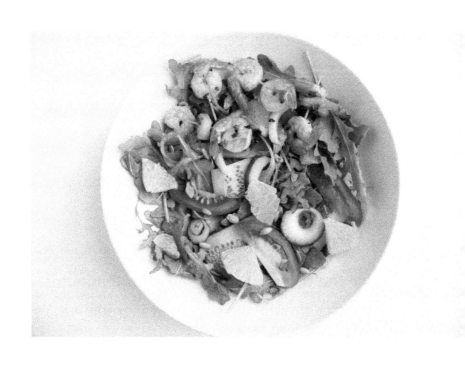

Eggplant and Tomato Stew

Prep time: 5 minutes I **Cooking time:** 20 minutes I

Servings: 4

Ingredients:

- 1 pound eggplants, roughly cubed
- 2 garlic cloves, minced
- 2 tablespoons olive oil
- 1 yellow onion, chopped
- 1 teaspoon sweet paprika
- ½ cup cilantro, chopped
- 14 ounces tomatoes, chopped
- 1 tablespoon cilantro, chopped

Directions:

1. Heat up a pan with the oil over medium-high heat, add the onion and the garlic and sauté for 2 minutes.
2. Add the eggplant and the other ingredients except the cilantro, bring to a simmer and cook for 18 minutes.
3. Divide into bowls and serve with the cilantro sprinkled on top.

Nutrition facts per serving: calories 343, fat 12.3, fiber 3.7, carbs 16.56, protein 7.2

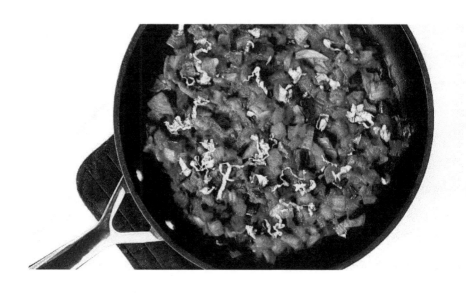

Parsley Beef and Peas Stew

Prep time: 10 minutes I **Cooking time:** 30 minutes I
Servings: 4

Ingredients:

- 1 and ¼ cups beef stock
- 1 yellow onion, chopped
- 1 tablespoon olive oil
- 2 cups peas
- 1 pound beef stew meat, cubed
- 1 cup tomatoes, chopped
- 1 cup scallions, chopped
- ¼ cup parsley, chopped
- Black pepper to the taste

Directions:

1. Heat up a pot with the oil over medium-high heat, add the onion and the meat and brown for 5 minutes.
2. Add the peas and the other ingredients, stir, bring to a simmer and cook over medium heat for 25 minutes more.
3. Divide the mix into bowls and serve for lunch.

Nutrition facts per serving: calories 487, fat 15.4, fiber 4.6, carbs 44.6, protein 17.8

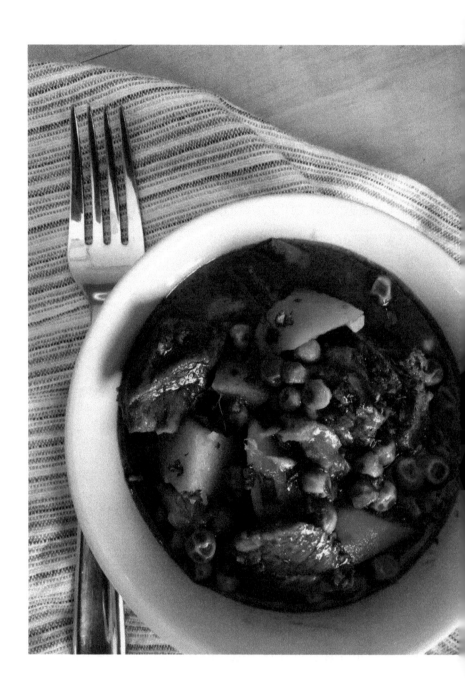

Lime Turkey Stew

Prep time: 5 minutes I **Cooking time:** 30 minutes I
Servings: 4

Ingredients:

- 2 tablespoons olive oil
- 1 turkey breast, skinless, boneless and cubed
- 1 cup beef stock
- 1 cup tomato puree
- ¼ teaspoon lime zest, grated
- 1 yellow onion, chopped
- 1 tablespoon sweet paprika
- 1 tablespoon cilantro, chopped
- 2 tablespoons lime juice
- ¼ teaspoon ginger, grated

Directions:

1. Heat up a pot with the oil over medium-high heat, add the onion and the meat and brown for 5 minutes.
2. Add the stock and the other ingredients, bring to a simmer and cook over medium heat for 25 minutes.
3. Divide the mix into bowls and serve for lunch.

Nutrition facts per serving: calories 150, fat 8.1, fibe

2.7, carbs 12, protein 9.5

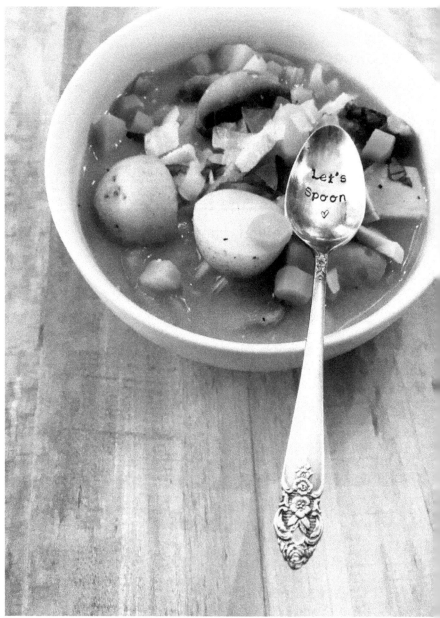

Beef and Black Beans Salad

Prep time: 10 minutes I **Cooking time:** 30 minutes I

Servings: 4

Ingredients:

- 1 pound beef stew meat, cut into strips
- 1 tablespoon sage, chopped
- 1 tablespoon olive oil
- A pinch of black pepper
- ½ teaspoon cumin, ground
- 2 cups cherry tomatoes, cubed
- 1 avocado, peeled, pitted and cubed
- 1 cup black beans, cooked and drained
- ½ cup green onions, chopped
- 2 tablespoons lime juice
- 2 tablespoons balsamic vinegar
- 2 tablespoons cilantro, chopped

Directions:

1. Heat up a pan with the oil over medium-high heat, add the meat and brown for 5 minutes.
2. Add the sage, black pepper and the cumin, toss and cook for 5 minutes more.
3. Add the rest of the ingredients, toss, reduce heat to medium and cook the mix for 20 minutes.

4. Divide the salad into bowls and serve for lunch

Nutrition facts per serving: calories 536, fat 21.4 fiber 12.5, carbs 40.4, protein 47

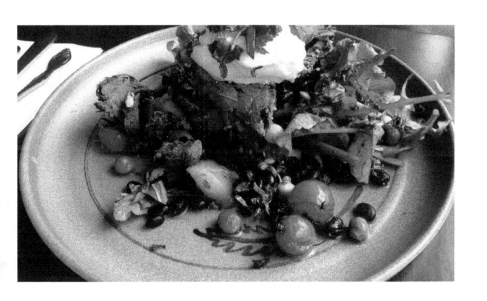

Squash and Peppers Mix

Prep time: 10 minutes I **Cooking time:** 20 minutes I

Servings: 4

Ingredients:

- 1 pound squash, peeled and roughly cubed
- 1 cup chicken stock
- 1 cup tomatoes, crushed
- 1 tablespoon olive oil
- 1 red onion, chopped
- 2 orange sweet peppers, chopped
- ½ cup quinoa
- ½ tablespoon chives, chopped

Directions:

1. Heat up a pot with the oil over medium heat add the onion, stir and sauté for 2 minutes.
2. Add the squash and the other ingredients, bring to a simmer, and cook for 15 minutes.
3. Stir the stew, divide into bowls and serve for lunch.

Nutrition facts per serving: calories 166, fat 5.3, fiber 4.7, carbs 26.3, protein 5.9

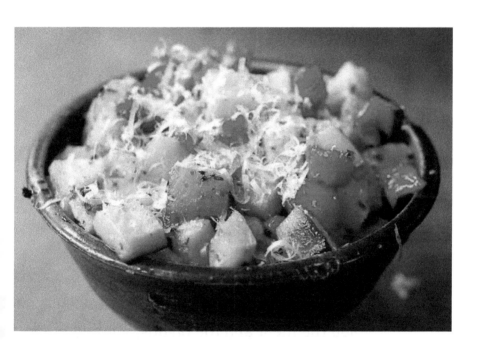

Beef, Green Onions and Peppers Mix

Prep time: 10 minutes I **Cooking time:** 20 minutes I

Servings: 4

Ingredients:

- 1 green cabbage head, shredded
- ¼ cup beef stock
- 2 tomatoes, cubed
- 2 yellow onions, chopped
- ¾ cup red bell peppers, chopped
- 1 tablespoon olive oil
- 1 pound beef, ground
- ¼ cup cilantro, chopped
- ¼ cup green onions, chopped
- ¼ teaspoon red pepper, crushed

Directions:

1. Heat up a pan with the oil over medium heat, add the meat and the onions, stir and brown for 5 minutes.
2. Add the cabbage and the other ingredients, toss, cook for 15 minutes, divide into bowls and serve for lunch.

Nutrition facts per serving: calories 328, fat 11, fiber 6.9, carbs 20.1, protein 38.3

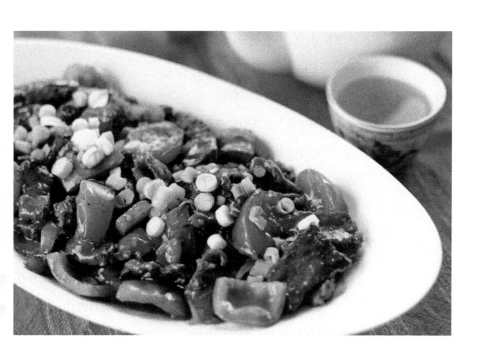

Pork, Green Beans and Tomato Stew

Prep time: 5 minutes I **Cooking time:** 8 hours and 10 minutes I **Servings:** 4

Ingredients:

- 1 pound pork stew meat, cubed
- 1 tablespoon olive oil
- ½ pound green beans, trimmed and halved
- 2 yellow onions, chopped
- 2 garlic cloves, minced
- 2 cups beef stock
- 8 ounces tomato sauce
- A pinch of black pepper
- A pinch of allspice, ground
- 1 tablespoon rosemary, chopped

Directions:

1. Heat up a pan with the oil over medium-high heat, add the meat, garlic and onion, stir and brown for 10 minutes.
2. Transfer this to a slow cooker, add the other ingredients as well, put the lid on and cook on Low for 8 hours.
3. Divide the stew into bowls and serve.

Nutrition facts per serving: calories 334, fat 14.8, fiber 4.4, carbs 13.3, protein 36.7

Garlic Turkey and Parsley

Prep time: 10 minutes I **Cooking time:** 30 minutes I

Servings: 4

Ingredients:

- 1 pound turkey breast, skinless, boneless and sliced
- 2 tablespoons olive oil
- 1 yellow onion, chopped
- ½ cup chicken stock
- 1 tablespoon basil, chopped
- 3 garlic cloves, minced
- ½ cup kalamata olives, pitted and sliced
- ¼ cup parsley, chopped

Directions:

1. Heat up a pan with the oil over medium heat, add the onion and the meat and brown for minutes.
2. Add the rest of the ingredients, toss, cover the pan and cook over medium heat for 25 minute more.
3. Divide everything between plates and serve fo lunch.

Nutrition facts per serving: calories 221, fat 2, fiber 4, carbs 7, protein 8

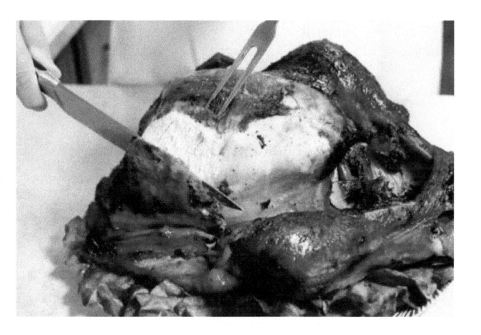

Thyme Chicken and Olives Stew

Prep time: 10 minutes I **Cooking time:** 40 minutes I

Servings: 4

Ingredients:

- 1 tablespoon olive oil
- 1 yellow onion, chopped
- 2 garlic cloves, minced
- 1 carrot, sliced
- 2 green chilies, chopped
- 1 teaspoon chili powder
- 1 zucchini, sliced
- ¼ cup tomato puree
- 1 pound chicken thighs, skinless, boneless and cubed
- A pinch of salt and black pepper
- ¼ teaspoon thyme, dried
- ¾ cup vegetable stock
- 2 tomatoes, cubed
- ¼ cup kalamata olives, pitted and halved
- 2 tablespoons basil, chopped

Directions:

1. Heat up a pot with the oil over medium heat add the onion and the garlic and sauté for minutes.

2. Add the meat and brown for 5 minutes more.

3. Add the rest of the ingredients, toss, bring the stew to a simmer, cook over medium heat for 30 minutes more.

4. Divide the stew into bowls and serve for lunch.

Nutrition facts per serving: calories 221, fat 2, fiber 3, carbs 8, protein 11

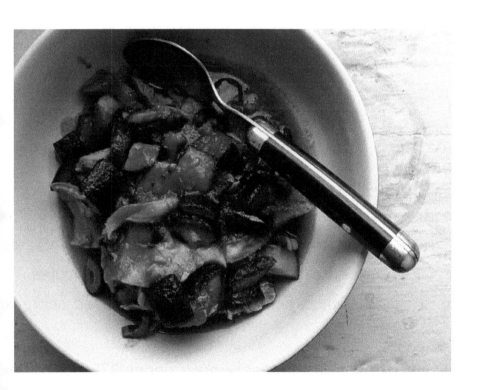

Turmeric and Paprika Chicken

Prep time: 10 minutes I **Cooking time:** 30 minutes I

Servings: 4

Ingredients:

- 1 pound chicken breast, skinless, boneless an
  sliced
- 1 tablespoon olive oil
- 2 tablespoons mustard
- 3 scallions, chopped
- Salt and black pepper to the taste
- ¼ cup chicken stock
- 4 chicken breasts, skinless and boneless
- ¼ teaspoon sweet paprika
- 1 teaspoon turmeric powder

Directions:

1. In a roasting pan, combine the chicken with th
   oil, the mustard and the other ingredients, tos
   and bake at 370 degrees F for 35 minutes.
2. Divide the mix between plates and serve fo
   lunch.

Nutrition facts per serving: calories 223, fat 8, fibe
1, carbs 3, protein 15

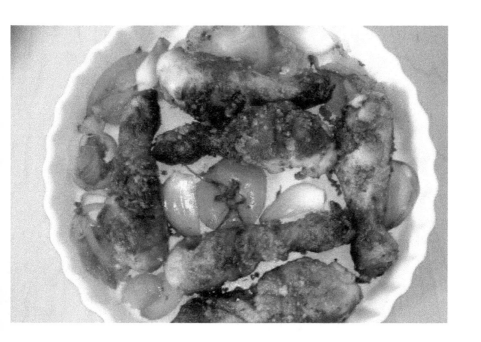

Balsamic Cabbage Bowls

Prep time: 5 minutes I **Cooking time:** 0 minutes I

Servings: 4

Ingredients:

- 2 avocados, pitted, peeled and cubed
- 2 cups red cabbage, shredded
- 2 tablespoons olive oil
- 3 scallions, chopped
- 1 tablespoon balsamic vinegar
- Salt and black pepper to the taste
- 1 tablespoon Dijon mustard
- ¼ cup lemon juice

Directions:

1. In a bowl, mix the cabbage with the avocado and the other ingredients, toss and serve for lunch right away.

Nutrition facts per serving: calories 211, fat 4, fiber 2, carbs 8, protein 7

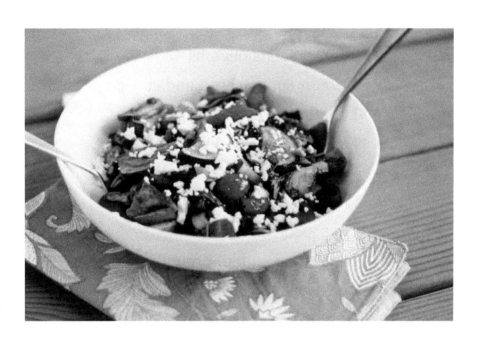

Mackerel and Apple Mix

Prep time: 10 minutes I **Cooking time:** 30 minutes I

Servings: 4

Ingredients:

- 4 mackerel fillets, boneless
- 1 yellow onion, sliced
- 2 tablespoons olive oil
- 1 green apple, cored and cut into wedges
- 2 tomatoes, cubed
- A pinch of salt and black pepper
- ¼ teaspoon turmeric powder
- ½ teaspoon oregano, chopped
- 1 teaspoon chili powder
- 1 teaspoon cumin, ground
- 3 tablespoons olive oil
- 3 garlic cloves, minced
- 3 tablespoons parsley, chopped

Directions:

1. In a roasting pan, combine the mackerel fillet with the onion, the oil, the apple and the other ingredients, toss gently and cook at 37 degrees F for 30 minutes.
2. Divide the mix between plates and serve for lunch.

Nutrition facts per serving: calories 441, fat 33.7, fiber 3.2, carbs 14.4, protein 22.4

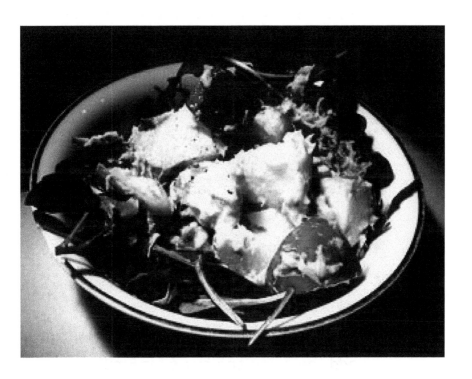

Fish and Avocado Stew

Prep time: 10 minutes I **Cooking time:** 30 minutes I

Servings: 4

Ingredients:

- 1 red onion, sliced
- 2 tablespoons olive oil
- 1 pound white fish fillets, boneless, skinless an
  cubed
- 1 avocado, pitted and chopped
- 1 tablespoon oregano, chopped
- 1 cup chicken stock
- 2 tomatoes, cubed
- 1 teaspoon sweet paprika
- A pinch of salt and black pepper
- 1 tablespoon parsley, chopped
- Juice of 1 lime

Directions:

1. Heat up a pot with the oil over medium hea
   add the onion and sauté for 5 minutes.
2. Add the fish, the avocado and the othe
   ingredients, toss, cook over medium heat fc
   25 minutes more, divide into bowls and serv
   for lunch.

Nutrition facts per serving: calories 390, fat 25.8, fiber 5.5, carbs 11.5, protein 30

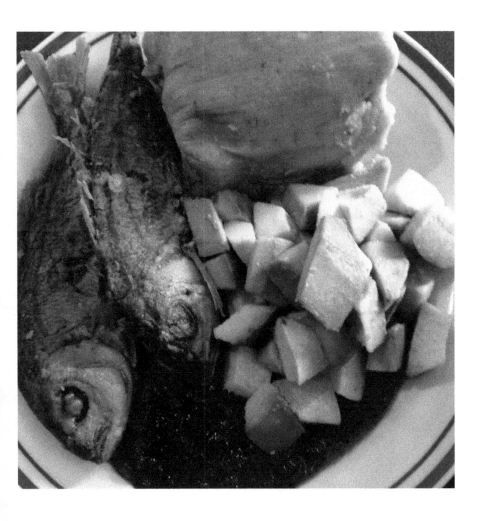

Lemon Chicken Mix

Prep time: 10 minutes I **Cooking time:** 30 minutes I

Servings: 4

Ingredients:

- 1 pound chicken breast, skinless, boneless and cubed
- 1 cup sun-dried tomatoes, chopped
- 1 yellow onion, chopped
- 2 tablespoons olive oil
- Juice of 1 lemon
- A pinch of salt and black pepper
- 1/3 cup pine nuts
- 1 tablespoon cilantro, chopped

Directions:

1. Heat up a pan with the oil over medium heat add the onion and the meat and brown for 5 minutes.
2. Add the sun-dried tomatoes and the other ingredients, toss, cook over medium heat for 25 minutes more, divide into bowls and serve for lunch.

Nutrition facts per serving: calories 288, fat 17.8 fiber 1.6, carbs 6.1, protein 26.4

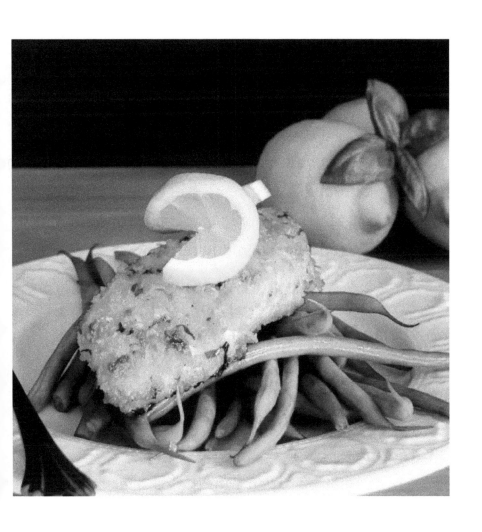

Chicken Stuffed Peppers

Prep time: 10 minutes I **Cooking time:** 45 minutes I

Servings: 4

Ingredients:

- 4 red bell peppers, tops cut off, deseeded
- 1 yellow onion, chopped
- 2 garlic cloves, minced
- 1 pound chicken breast, skinless, boneless and ground
- 1 tablespoon oregano, chopped
- 1 tablespoon lime juice
- ¼ teaspoon cumin, ground
- ½ teaspoon oregano, dried
- ¼ teaspoon turmeric powder
- A pinch of salt and black pepper
- 2 tablespoons olive oil
- 1 cup tomato puree

Directions:

1. Heat up a pan with the oil over medium heat, add the onion, the garlic and the chicken meat and brown for 5 minutes.
2. Add the rest of the ingredients except the bell peppers and the tomato puree, stir, cook for minutes more and take off the heat.

3. Stuff the peppers with this mix, arrange them in a roasting pan, pour the tomato puree over them and bake at 370 degrees F for 30 minutes.
4. Divide the peppers between plates and serve for lunch.

Nutrition facts per serving: calories 272, fat 10.5, fiber 4.1, carbs 19.6, protein 26.9

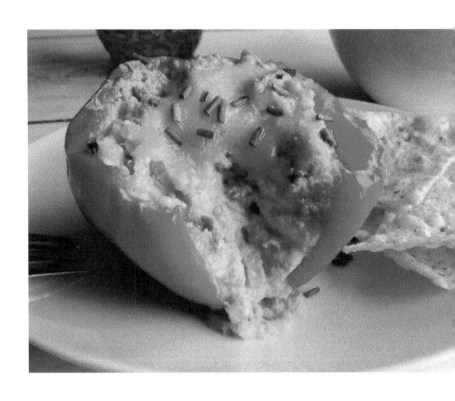

Coconut Veggie Soup

Prep time: 10 minutes I **Cooking time:** 30 minutes I
Servings: 4

Ingredients:

- 1 yellow onion, chopped
- 1 pound zucchinis, chopped
- 1 green chili pepper, chopped
- 1 tablespoon olive oil
- A pinch of salt and black pepper
- 4 garlic cloves, minced
- 4 cups vegetable stock
- 1 cup coconut cream
- 1 tablespoon parsley, chopped

Directions:

1. Heat up a pot with the oil over medium-high heat, add the onion, the chili pepper and the garlic and sauté for 5 minutes.
2. Add the zucchinis and the rest of the ingredients except the cream, bring to a simmer and cook over medium heat for 25 minutes more.
3. Add the cream, blend the soup using an immersion blender, divide into bowls and serve.

Nutrition facts per serving: calories 180, fat 2, fibe
2, carbs 7, protein 5

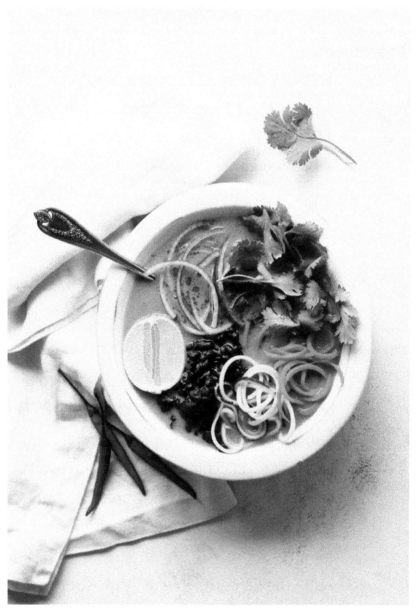

Parsley Shrimp Soup

Prep time: 5 minutes I **Cooking time:** 25 minutes I
Servings: 4

Ingredients:

- 2 tablespoons olive oil
- 1 yellow onion, chopped
- 4 cups chicken stock
- Juice of 1 lime
- 1 pound shrimp, peeled and deveined
- ½ cup coconut cream
- ½ pound broccoli florets
- 1 tablespoon parsley, chopped

Directions:

1. Heat up a pot with the oil over medium heat, add the onion and sauté for 5 minutes.
2. Add the shrimp and the other ingredients, toss, bring to a simmer and cook over medium heat for 20 minutes more.
3. Ladle the soup into bowls and serve for lunch.

Nutrition facts per serving: calories 190, fat 3, fiber 2, carbs 6, protein 8

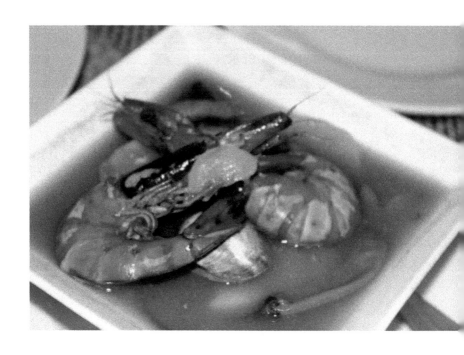

Turkey and Zucchini Mix

Prep time: 10 minutes I **Cooking time:** 30 minutes I

Servings: 4

Ingredients:

- 1 yellow onion, chopped
- 1 pound turkey breast, skinless, boneless and cubed
- 2 tablespoons olive oil
- 2 garlic cloves, minced
- 1 zucchini, sliced
- 1 cup coconut cream
- A pinch of sea salt and black pepper

Directions:

1. Heat up a pan with the oil over medium heat, add the onion and the garlic and sauté for 5 minutes.
2. Add the meat and brown for 5 minutes more.
3. Add the rest of the ingredients, toss, bring to a simmer and cook over medium heat for 20 minutes more.
4. Divide the mix into bowls and serve for lunch.

Nutrition facts per serving: calories 200, fat 4, fiber 2, carbs 14, protein 7

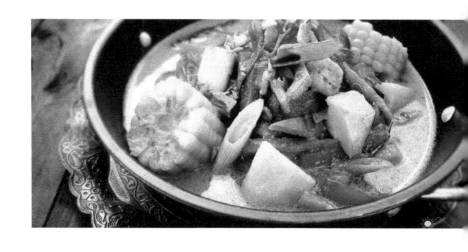

Potato and Spinach Soup

Prep time: 10 minutes I **Cooking time:** 35 minutes I

Servings: 4

Ingredients:

- 1 yellow onion, chopped
- 1 tablespoon olive oil
- 3 sweet potatoes, peeled and cubed
- 5 cups chicken stock
- 1 cup baby spinach
- 1 tomato, cubed
- A pinch of sea salt and black pepper

Directions:

1. Heat up a pot with the oil over medium heat, add the onion and sauté for 5 minutes.
2. Add the sweet potatoes and the other ingredients, toss, bring to a simmer and cook over medium heat for 30 minutes more.
3. Ladle the soup into bowls and serve for lunch.

Nutrition facts per serving: calories 200, fat 8.2, fiber 2, carbs 11.6, protein 8

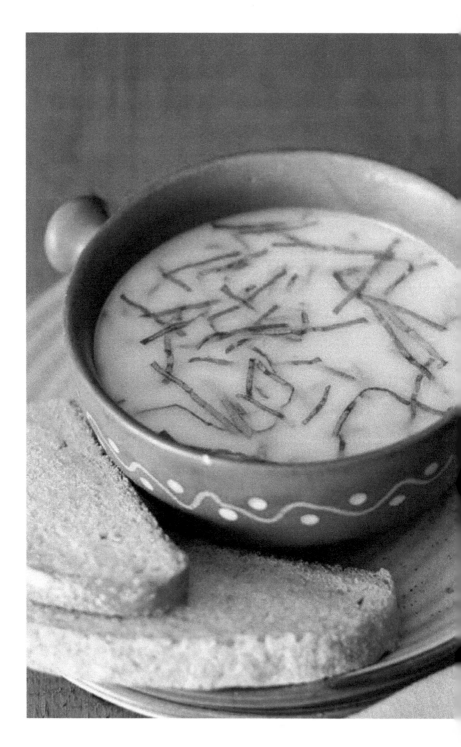

Artichoke and Tomato Soup

Prep time: 5 minutes I **Cooking time:** 30 minutes I

Servings: 4

Ingredients:

- 2 tablespoons olive oil
- 2 yellow onions, chopped
- 2 cups artichoke hearts, halved
- A pinch of salt and black pepper
- 5 cups vegetable stock
- 2 tomatoes, cubed
- ¼ teaspoon turmeric powder
- 1 teaspoon cumin, ground
- 1 tablespoon rosemary, chopped
- 1 tablespoon tomato paste

Directions:

1. Heat up a pot with the oil over medium-high heat, add the onions and sauté for 5 minutes.
2. Add the artichokes and the other ingredients, toss, bring to a simmer and cook over medium heat for 25 minutes more.
3. Ladle the soup into bowls and serve.

Nutrition facts per serving: calories 200, fat 4, fiber 4, carbs 12, protein 8

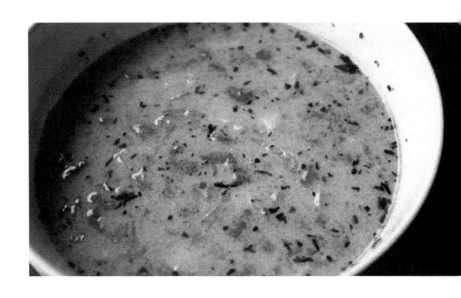

Cayenne Chicken and Shrimp

Prep time: 5 minutes I **Cooking time:** 20 minutes I

Servings: 4

Ingredients:

- 1 yellow onion, chopped
- 2 tablespoons olive oil
- 1 pound chicken breast, skinless, boneless and cubed
- ½ pound shrimp, peeled and deveined
- ½ cup chicken stock
- A pinch of sea salt and black pepper
- ¼ teaspoon cayenne pepper
- ¼ teaspoon turmeric powder
- 1 teaspoon sweet paprika
- ½ tablespoon cilantro, chopped

Directions:

1. Heat up a pan with the oil over medium heat, add the onion and the meat and cook for 10 minutes.
2. Add the shrimp and the other ingredients, toss, cook over medium heat for 10 minutes more, divide into bowls and serve for lunch.

Nutrition facts per serving: calories 280, fat 3, fibe
3, carbs 6, protein 7

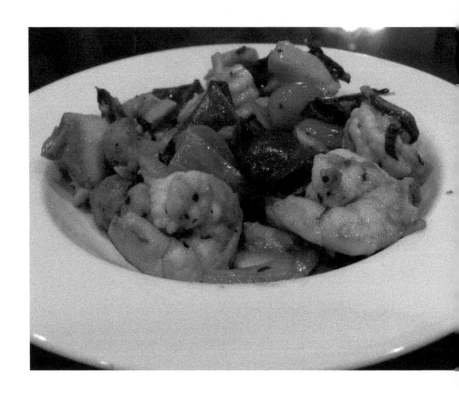

Kale Stew

Prep time: 10 minutes I **Cooking time:** 25 minutes I

Servings: 4

Ingredients:

- 1 pound tomatoes, roughly cubed
- ½ pound kale, torn
- 1 yellow onion, chopped
- 1 tablespoon olive oil
- 1 cup tomato puree
- A pinch of cayenne pepper
- 1 teaspoon cumin powder
- 1 teaspoon chili powder
- 1 teaspoon cumin, ground
- A pinch of salt and black pepper
- ½ tablespoon cilantro, chopped

Directions:

1. Heat up a pot with the oil over medium heat, add the onion and sauté for 5 minutes.
2. Add the tomatoes, the kale and the other ingredients, toss, bring to a simmer and cook over medium heat for 20 minutes.
3. Divide the stew into bowls and serve for lunch.

Nutrition facts per serving: calories 210, fat 5, fibe
5, carbs 14, protein 8

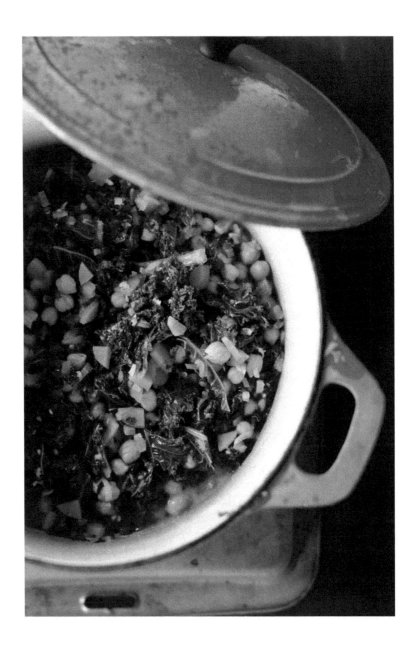

Lime Shrimp

Prep time: 10 minutes I **Cooking time:** 20 minutes I
Servings: 4

Ingredients:

- 1 pound shrimp, peeled and deveined
- 4 scallions, chopped
- 1 teaspoon sweet paprika
- 1 tablespoon olive oil
- Juice of 1 lime
- Zest of 1 lime, grated
- A pinch of salt and black pepper
- 2 tablespoons parsley, chopped

Directions:

1. Heat up a pan with the oil over medium heat, add the scallions and sauté for 5 minutes.
2. Add the shrimp and the other ingredients, toss, cook over medium heat for 15 minutes more, divide into bowls and serve.

Nutrition facts per serving: calories 172, fat 5.5, fiber 0.7, carbs 3.3, protein 26.2

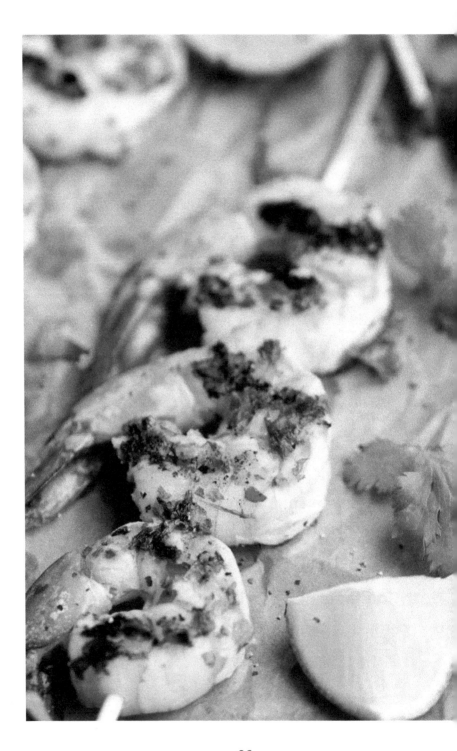

Lemon Cod

Prep time: 10 minutes I **Cooking time:** 20 minutes I

Servings: 4

Ingredients:

- 1 tablespoon olive oil
- 2 shallots, chopped
- 4 cod fillets, boneless and skinless
- 2 garlic cloves, minced
- 2 tablespoons lemon juice
- 1 cup chicken stock
- A pinch of salt and black pepper

Directions:

1. Heat up a pan with the oil over medium-high heat, add the shallots and the garlic and sauté for 5 minutes.
2. Add the cod and the other ingredients, cook everything for 15 minutes more, divide between plates and serve for lunch.

Nutrition facts per serving: calories 130, fat 4.7, fiber 0.1, carbs 1.7, protein 20.5

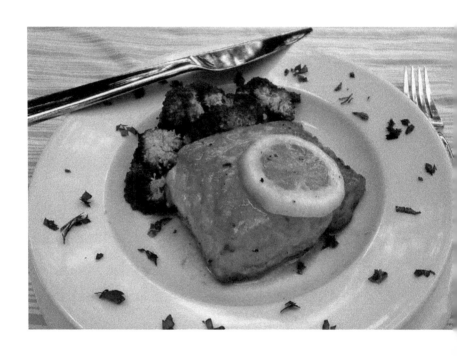

Oregano Chicken and Tomato Mix

Prep time: 5 minutes I **Cooking time:** 30 minutes I

Servings: 4

Ingredients:

- 1 pound chicken breast, skinless, boneless and roughly cubed
- 1 yellow onion, chopped
- 1 tablespoon olive oil
- 1 tablespoon lime juice
- 2 garlic cloves, minced
- 1 teaspoon turmeric powder
- 1 teaspoon chili powder
- 1 teaspoon sweet paprika
- A pinch of salt and black pepper
- 1 cup cherry tomatoes, halved
- 1 tablespoon oregano, chopped
- 1 tablespoon chives, chopped
- 1 red chili pepper, chopped

Directions:

1. Heat up a pan with the oil over medium heat, add the onion, garlic and the meat and cook for 10 minutes.
2. Add the lime juice, turmeric and the other ingredients, toss, cook over medium heat for

20 minutes more, divide into bowls and serve warm for lunch.

Nutrition facts per serving: calories 210, fat 3, fiber 2, carbs 13, protein 8

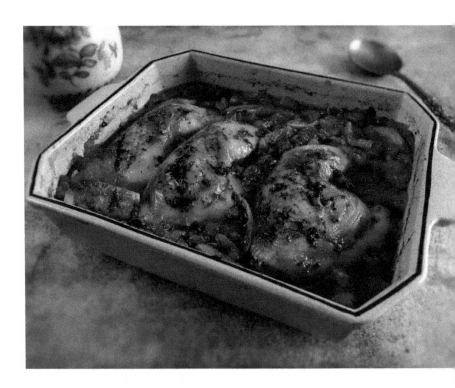

Salmon and Tomato Sauce

Prep time: 5 minutes I **Cooking time:** 25 minutes I
Servings: 4

Ingredients:

- 4 salmon fillets, boneless
- 1 yellow onion, chopped
- 2 tablespoons olive oil
- 1 cup red cabbage, shredded
- 1 red bell pepper, chopped
- 1 tablespoon rosemary, chopped
- 1 tablespoon coriander, ground
- 1 cup tomato sauce
- A pinch of sea salt and black pepper

Directions:

1. Heat up a pan with the oil over medium heat, add the onion and sauté for 5 minutes.
2. Add the fish and sear it for 2 minutes on each side.
3. Add the cabbage and the remaining ingredients, toss, cook over medium heat for 20 minutes more, divide between plates and serve.

Nutrition facts per serving: calories 210, fat 4, fiber 5, carbs 12, protein 8

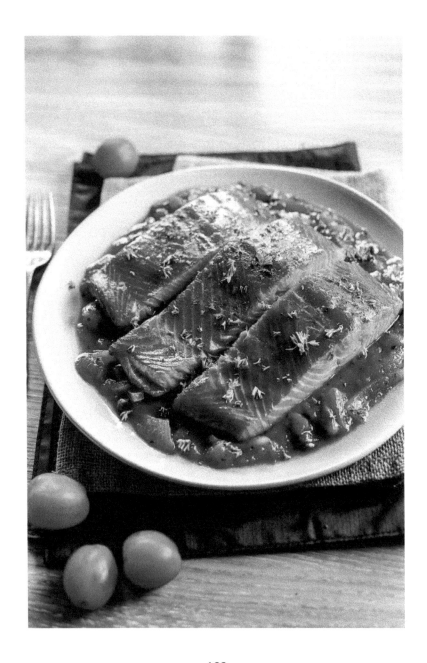

Burritos

Prep time: 5 minutes I **Cooking time:** 12 minutes I **Servings:** 4

Ingredients:

- 1 cup black beans, cooked
- 1 green bell pepper, chopped
- 1 carrots, peeled and grated
- 1 tablespoon olive oil
- 1 red onion, sliced
- ½ cup corn
- 1 cup cheddar, shredded
- 6 corn tortillas
- 1 cup Greek yogurt

Directions:

1. Heat up a pan with the oil over medium heat, add the onion and sauté for 2 minutes.
2. Add the beans, carrot, bell pepper and the corn, stir, and cook for 10 minutes more.
3. Arrange the tortillas on a working surface, divide the beans mix on each, also divide the cheese and the yogurt, roll and serve for lunch.

Nutrition facts per serving: calories 451, fat 7.5, fiber 13.8, carbs 78.2, protein 20.9

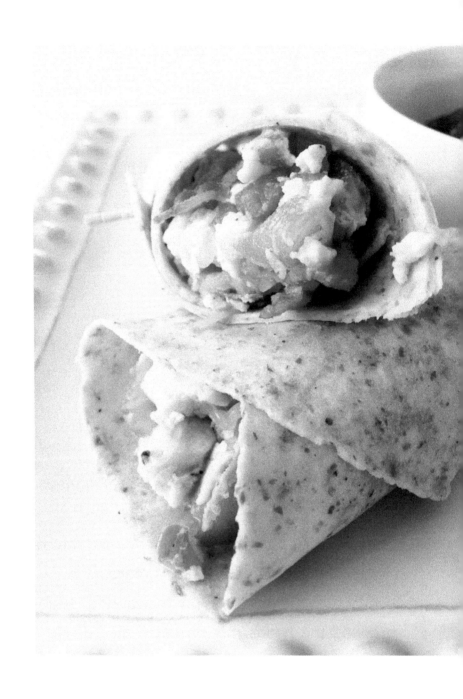

Chicken with Spinach and Mango

Prep time: 10 minutes I **Cooking time:** 20 minutes I
Servings: 4

Ingredients:

- 2 chicken breasts, skinless, boneless and cubed
- ¼ cup chicken stock
- ½ cup celery, chopped
- 1 cup baby spinach
- 1 mango, peeled, and cubed
- 2 spring onions, chopped
- 1 tablespoon olive oil
- 1 teaspoon thyme, dried
- ¼ teaspoon garlic powder
- A pinch of black pepper

Directions:

1. Heat up a pan with the oil over medium-high heat, add the spring onions and the chicken and brown for 5 minutes.
2. Add the celery and the other ingredients except the spinach, toss and cook for 12 minutes more.
3. Add the spinach, toss, cook for 2-3 minutes, divide everything between plates and serve.

Nutrition facts per serving: calories 221, fat 9.1, fibe 2, carbs 14.1, protein 21.5

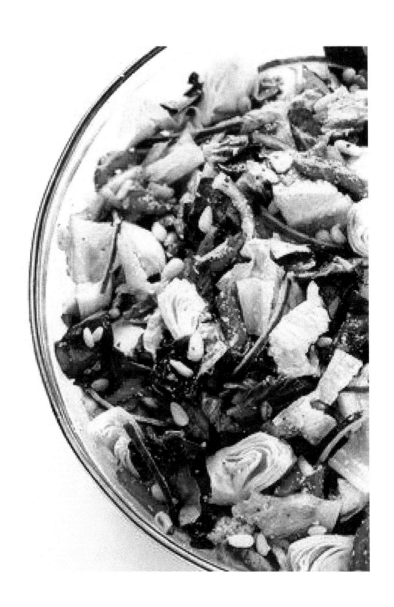

Veggie Cakes

Prep time: 10 minutes I **Cooking time:** 10 minutes I
Servings: 4

Ingredients:

- 2 garlic cloves, minced
- 15 ounces chickpeas, cooked
- 1 teaspoon chili powder
- 1 teaspoon cumin, ground
- 1 egg
- 1 tablespoon olive oil
- 1 tablespoon lime juice
- 1 tablespoon lime zest, grated
- 1 tablespoon cilantro, chopped

Directions:

1. In a blender, combine the chickpeas with the garlic and the other ingredients except the egg and pulse well.
2. Shape medium cakes out of this mix.
3. Heat up a pan with the oil over medium-high heat, add the chickpeas cakes, cook for 5 minutes on each side, divide between plates and serve for lunch with a side salad.

Nutrition facts per serving: calories 441, fat 11.3
fiber 19, carbs 66.4, protein 22.2

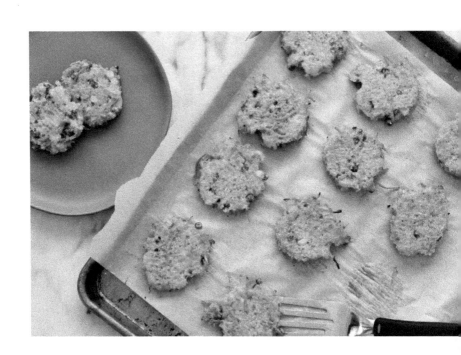

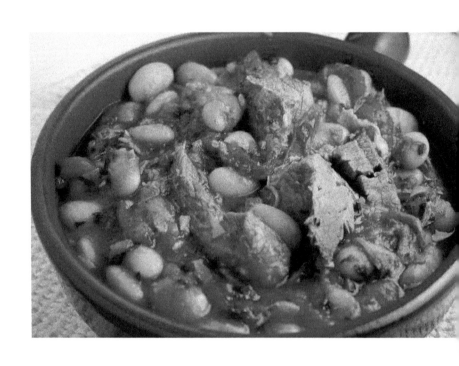

Lightning Source UK Ltd.
Milton Keynes UK
UKHW020812110621
385331UK00004B/113